LOW-SALI
FOOD DICTIONARY

The World's Most Comprehensive Low-Salicylate Ingredient Dictionary: Take It Wherever You Go!

BY THE SALICYLATE HEROES

Copyright: The Salicylate Heroes 2021

All rights reserved. No part of this guide may be reproduced in any form without permission in writing from the publisher except in the case of brief quotations embodied in critical articles or reviews.

LEGAL & DISCLAIMER

The information contained in this book is not designed to replace or take the place of any form of medicine or professional medical advice. The information in this book has been provided for educational and entertainment purposes only.

You need to consult a professional medical practitioner in order to ensure you are both healthy enough and able to make use of this information. Always consult your professional medical practitioner before undertaking any new dietary regime, and particularly after reading this book.

The information contained in this book has been compiled from sources deemed reliable, and it is accurate to the best of the Author's knowledge; however, the Author cannot guarantee its accuracy and validity and cannot be held liable for any errors or omissions.

You must consult your doctor or get professional medical advice before using any suggested information in this book.

Upon using the information contained in this book, you agree to hold harmless the Author, and Publisher, from and against any damages, costs, and expenses, including any legal fees potentially resulting from the application of any of the information provided by this guide. This disclaimer applies to any damages or injury caused by the use and application, whether directly or indirectly, of any advice or information presented, whether for breach of contract, tort, negligence, personal injury, criminal intent, or under any other cause of action. You agree to accept all risks of using the information presented inside this book.

INTRODUCTION

Congratulations on choosing this book. We wrote it because we suffer from food intolerances, including salicylate issues, ourselves.

If you have the same problem, you've probably experienced a similar level of frustration with much of the information out there conflicting with other sources.

Here's what often happens.

One list will tell you a food is low in salicylates while another will rank it as high in salicylates.

That just ends up being confusing for everyone! So we decided to take the world's best and most trusted salicylate lists and guides and compile the information into one easy-to-consult guide.

Trust us, it's been quite the process.
Even as we wrote this guide, we noticed that many of the top lists massively disagree on salicylate content in food.

As we know now, that's the nature of salicylate issues. Everybody reacts differently, and foods even show up differently depending on the salicylates present.

That's why we wanted to write this list. We believe it is the most comprehensive out there, and where there is debate, we have deferred to many of these top sources. With all that said, there will be areas you disagree on and that is why a) approach any new food with caution, and b) always consult your medical practitioner before making any dietary changes.

We know this list will never be definitive, and we will continue to refine it as more information becomes available.

MORE ON SALICYLATES

This book is not for everyone. As the *Healthline* reports, there's no reason to avoid salicylates unless you think you might have a sensitivity or intolerance to them.

Salicylate intolerance is not as common as lactose or gluten intolerance, or even lectin or oxalate intolerance. However there's no doubt that it's a serious problem for many.

We want to be clear, we take salicylate intolerance incredibly seriously. We've seen how people can turn their health around once they start to focus on it.

So let's briefly look into the science of salicylates and what they actually are.

Salicylates are chemicals. They are found naturally (think food and plants) and can be produced synthetically too (think medications, personal hygiene products and other items). They can cause adverse reactions to those who are intolerant, with a sensitivity linked to many different symptoms that can make it hard to identify.

Consuming excessive amounts of salicylates can result in

adverse reactions in anyone, although most people can safely eat foods that contain them on a regular basis.

For who have an intolerance though, it's a different story.

Why?

Scientific research has found that some people have a reduced ability to metabolize and excrete them properly.

One such study in *Inflammopharmacology* found that this may be due to an overproduction of leukotrienes which have been associated with conditions like inflammatory bowel disease, rheumatoid arthritis, and asthma. It's caused by an enzyme called cyclooxygenase which aids in regulating the production of leukotrienes.

All fairly technical, admittedly.

The key though, if you have salicylate issues, is to limiting these side effects. They include sleeping disorders, skin rashes, and gastrointestinal symptoms, and they are the reason we wrote this book. And the way to avoid them, we believe, is primarily by avoiding high salicylate foods.

That makes it important to have as definitive a source as possible to consult. That's why we decided to compile the most reliable, science-based salicylate information and food lists so that they can be found in one guide that makes it easy to consult. We've brought all the available information together into this one guide.

We've also included a short section at the end of this dictionary on non-food items - *Household Cleaning Products, Chemicals, Personal Care Items and Medicines.*

One of the key things to remember is that it's impossible to avoid all salicylates and it's not advisable to try. The goal should be to reduce the level of salicylates in your body to limit or potentially eliminate unwanted symptoms and maintain that state so that they don't reappear. In conjunction with your practitioner, hopefully this will be a temporary, not permanent solution.

Foods that are high in salicylates are anti-inflammatory and can lower the risk of inflammatory diseases like arthritis and even some cancers as research published in the *Food & Journal* revealed. Plus, many herbs, spices, fruits and vegetables that are high in salicylates benefit one's health with potent plant compounds, minerals and vitamins. So eventually, you'll want to try and reintroduce some of these foods. But that is for another day.

All of the above means means you should consult with your practitioner to determine the correct course for you before using this dictionary. Please keep in mind that materials and resources like this book are no substitute for medical advice and not intended as such.

Without further ado, let's get straight on to our salicylate food dictionary.

HOW TO USE THIS LOW SALICYLATE FOOD DICTIONARY

This book works exactly like other dictionaries. Look for a food, drink or ingredient alphabetically (or use the search function if viewing on a device).

Once you find what you are looking for, it is scored between 1 and 5 for salicylate levels based on careful analysis of the world's best sources (listed below) for salicylate content.

Some online titles detail either cup size, serving size or the precise amount of mg of salicylate levels per 100 g. That can be useful, but we get hungry, which means one of our servings might be three of someone else's.

We've made it more straightforward in this book. We've consulted those sites, and each food gets a score. The higher the score, the better it is for your low salicylate diet.

- 5 is best (indicates good choice for a low-salicylate diet as per our sources)

- 1 is worst (indicates poor choice for a low-salicylate diet as per our sources)

That means when following a low-salicylate diet, 5 is best and 1 is worst. Initially, you'll aim to consume more "5" foods and cut out "1" foods. As time goes on, with the help of a skilled practitioner, you would look to address the root cause of your salicylate issues and perhaps reintroduce foods gradually as you're able to, in order to maximize the nutrition in your diet.

We decided on a scoring system between 1 and 5 as many food sources only group foods into 'high' or 'low' salicylate (or 'bad' and 'good,' and we feel there is considerably more nuance to food intolerances, allergies and analysis. Respected sites can disagree on major foods, so we've tried to reflect that in our dictionary.

At this point, we probably need to insert a disclaimer. Our aim is to help you to heal from salicylate issues so that you can live a healthy, balanced life in every aspect.

This book has been a labor of love, and it has been a challenge (as mentioned) to put together as our major sources disagree so often about salicylate content. That's exactly why we wrote it, and why you must consult your doctor or get professional medical advice before using any information suggested in this book. Everyone has a unique and individual body chemistry and should take advice on salicylate issues.

Keep this book close by when you cook or eat out, and dip in and out whenever you need to check if something is low salicylate. We also encourage you to explore the section at the end of this dictionary entitled *Household Cleaning Products, Chemicals, Personal Care Items and Medicines*. This may help you further on your journey to a healthy, low-salicylate life.

SOURCES

We have consulted many sources in the course of our research in order to compile the most comprehensive, accurate list as possible. We highly recommend that you take advantage of these outstanding studies, research papers, links and sites in your further research on salicylates.

- ResearchGate - A systematic review of salicylates in foods: Estimated daily intake of a Scottish population
  https://www.researchgate.net/publication/50197171_A_systematic_review_of_salicylates_in_foods_Estimated_daily_intake_of_a_Scottish_population

- Diet vs Disease – Salicylate Intolerance: The Complete Guide + List of Foods
  https://www.dietvsdisease.org/salicylate-intolerance/

- Journal of the American Dietetic Association – Salicylates in foods
  https://www.slhd.nsw.gov.au/rpa/allergy/research/salicylatesinfoods.pdf

- Food & Function – Natural salicylates: foods, functions

and disease prevention
https://pubmed.ncbi.nlm.nih.gov/21879102/

- Dr. Richard Coleman, Millhouse Integrative Medical Centre – MMC Fact Sheet 908 Salicylate Content of Foods
http://www.millhousemedical.co.nz/files/docs/factsheet_8_salicylates_in_foods.pdf

- Journal of the American Dietetic Association - Are there foods that should be avoided if a patient is sensitive to salicylates?
https://pubmed.ncbi.nlm.nih.gov/20497789/

- Nutrients journal – Effectiveness of Personalized Low Salicylate Diet in the Management of Salicylates Hypersensitive Patients: Interventional Study
https://www.ncbi.nlm.nih.gov/pmc/articles/PMC8003553/

- Healthline – Salicylate Sensitivity: Causes, Symptoms and Foods to Avoid
https://www.healthline.com/nutrition/salicylate-sensitivity

- Healthline – Should You Avoid Salicylates?
https://www.healthline.com/nutrition/salicylate-sensitivity#TOC_TITLE_HDR_7

- Food Can Make You Ill Food List - https://www.foodcanmakeyouill.co.uk/salicylate-in-food.html

- WebMD – High Salicylate Foods - https://www.webmd.com/diet/high-salicylate-foods#1

THE SALICYLATE FOOD DICTIONARY

- 5 is best (indicates good for a low-salicylate diet as per sources above)
- 1 is worst (indicates poor choice for low-salicylate diet as per sources above)

Acerola: 2

A fruit similar to a cherry, also red when it's ripe, acerola is a rich source of vitamin C and contains many minerals and other vitamins like beta-carotene.

There isn't much information available on the amount of salicylates acerola specifically contains (welcome to the frustrations of salicylate issues). The Go Figure website notes acerola may cause salicylate issues in sensitive individuals. and we believe as cherries contain a high content, it's best to avoid or limit consumption.

Agave syrup: 3

While honey and most sweets tend to be high in salicylates, agave syrup are thought to contain a more moderate amount.

The way that it's processed, using heat and enzymes, destroys health-promoting benefits from the agave plant.

Limit your use and proceed with caution.

Alcohol: 2

Alcoholic beverages like beer, wine, and spirits such as rum and sherry tend to contain a high level of salicylates.

Champagne and sparkling wine are on the higher end, with Drambuie containing one of the highest levels for a liqueur. Dry white wines have a lower amount while beer and ale can range anywhere from .32 to 1.26 per 100 g.

Of course, there are also the other negative health effects of alcohol to consider.

Algae: 3

There is not a lot of information available related to salicylates and algae. However, spirulina, a blue-green algae known for its many health benefits has been well-documented in studies to contain an active compound called C-phycocyanin.

This component was shown to significantly reduce tinnitus secondary to high amounts of salicylates which may indicate that it is a low salicylate food.

This is not conclusive though. We have rated it a 3 rather than 5; proceed with caution.

Almond: 2

Almonds are thought to contain a high level of salicylates.

They do have other health positives - they aid in the regeneration of the nervous system and have many other benefits. They are a good supply of protein and iron, and beneficial for vegans and vegetarians; however, when limiting salicylates, it's best to consume a small amount, just one to three rather than a handful.

Anchovies: 5

Anchovies are considered to be low in salicylates and rich in omega-3 fatty acids which offer powerful benefits for heart health, including reducing blood pressure and triglyceride levels.

They also contain a high level of B3 and selenium.

Apple: 2

Salicylate content can vary wildly with apples, so it is worth proceeding with caution.

The amount of salicylates in apples is thought to depend on the type of apple. And people wonder why salicylate intolerance is confusing!

Golden and Red Delicious are thought to contain the least at .1-.25 milligrams (mg) per 100 grams (g), while Granny Smith have the highest level at .5 – 1 mg.

Be aware that some sources, including WebMD, recommend

avoiding apples altogether so proceed carefully.

Apple cider vinegar: 2

Opinion is split. Apple cider vinegar in foods may not cause a problem; however, taking it as a supplement and/or drinking it straight is not advised due to the high level of salicylates.

The website Allergenics notes;

Sauces and Condiments: most commercial or store-bought gravies, sauces and pastes (eg. tomato paste, worcester sauce, gravy mix), jams, marmalades, fruit/mint/honey flavouring, chewing gum, white and cider vinegars

Apricot: 1

Apricots are thought to have a very high level of salicylates with over 1 mg per 100 g of the fruit.

While they are rich in vitamin A, beta-carotene, and other carotenoids, when following a low-salicylate diet, carrots are your better bet for these nutrients.

And dried apricot may be even worse.

The website *Food Can Make You Ill* provides a comprehensive breakdown of an Australian study (Anne R Swain et al. Salicylates in Food. Journal of the American Dietetic Association Vol. 85:8 1985). It puts dried apricots and dates in its 'Extremely high amounts of salicylates' section.

Artichokes: 3

Artichokes, whether they're the French or Jerusalem type, are moderately high in salicylates.

According to *Healthline*, compared to other vegetables they contain some of the highest levels at .5 to 1 mg per 100 g.

However, if you eat them by gently scraping off the tender bits at the bottom of the leaf, closing your teeth on it and pulling the leaf outward, rather than eating the entire heart, you may be able to consume that small amount. (This sounds a little complicated for us!)

Artificial sweeteners: 1

Plain artificial sweeteners are thought to have a low level of salicylates; however, these additives are best avoided as they can trigger symptoms similar to the adverse effects of salicylates depending on the individual.

Additionally, they are well-documented scientifically for the potential to cause harm to one's health, including weight gain and certain cancers.

Asparagus: 3

We have looked at two types of asparagus. Canned asparagus is richer in salicylates with one 1 mg per 100 g. If you're going to consume it, choose fresh asparagus. There is some conflicting information as to the exact level of salicylates it contains, rated low to moderate depending on the source.

Most reliable studies have noted that it has a low amount with levels below .25 per 100 g, but not all.

Asparagus is high in folic acid and a good source of vitamins A, B6, C, as well as potassium and fiber.

Aubergine: 2

More commonly known as eggplant, aubergine is a well-known nightshade vegetable that's jam-packed with nutrients, but it also has a higher level of salicylates than many other vegetables at .5 to 1 mg per 100 g.

If you consume, do so only in limited amounts. Some diets such as the Bulletproof Diet consider Aubergine to be inflammatory.

Avocado: 2

Avocados tend to be on the list of foods to avoid for those with a salicylate sensitivity.

Bamboo shoots: 4

All reliable sources list bamboo shoots as having a low or negligible amount of salicylates.

Highly nutritious, they're a good source of vitamins B6 and E, fiber, and copper.

Banana: 5

Lots of fruits are frustratingly high on salicylates, but not bananas. That's why we picked them for the front cover of this guide.

Bananas tend to be very low in salicylates with less than .1 mg per 100 g. They contain a significant amount of vitamin B6 as well as potassium and other nutrients.

Barley: 4

Barley isn't gluten-free, but it is considered a healthy whole grain that contains only a negligible amount of salicylates.

To avoid additives (which might change the salicylate content), use it as an ingredient in a homemade bread.

Barley malt, malt: 1

See "Malt"

Basil: 5

Our research suggests basil is a herb that contains one of the highest levels of salicylates.

While the number of milligrams is not available due to limited research, avoid or proceed with caution, using only a small amount.

Beans: 4

Beans and salicylates are a little complicated. When is it ever not complicated with salicylates?

Most beans contain only trace amounts; however French beans may have up to .25 mg per 100 g. Avoid or limit broad and fava beans which have a higher level.

Beef: 4

See "Meat"

Beer: 4

See "Alcohol."

Beetroot: 3

It is difficult to definitely rate beetroot. We have come across a lot of conflicting research. Based on this divergence of opinion we have given it a "3" and believe it may be best to avoid canned beetroot and choose fresh, proceeding with caution.

Let's explain in a little more detail.

There is some debate as to the level of salicylates in beetroot. According to research published in the *Journal of the American Dietetic Association,* fresh beets have just .18 mg per 100 g. Canned beets are higher, with a moderate amount of up to .49 mg per 100 g.

When we dig into our sources, Millhouse Medical Centre categorizes beets in general as moderate, while Drugs.com puts beetroot in the "high" category, and the other lists also cannot quite agree.

So... as always, proceed carefully and find your individual tolerance level.

Bell pepper (hot): 3

Hot peppers are very high in salicylates although the

capsaicin they contain may reduce adverse effects.

Consume minimally until you know how your body will react.

Avoid sweet peppers which contain a high level of salicylates without the capsaicin.

Bell pepper (sweet): 1

Sweet bell peppers also have a high level of salicylates. Avoid sweet peppers which contain a high level of salicylates without the capsaicin.

Bison: 5

Meat is generally salicylate-free, and bison can be a good alternative to beef as it contains less saturated fat and is lower in calories.

While it's more expensive, grass-fed bison is best. Traditionally farmed options cost less but have a different nutritional profile as multiple studies have noted.

Bivalves (mussels, oyster, clams, scallops): 5

Have you ever heard of the term bivalves? That's probably not what you call oysters or mussels when you order them at a restaurant, but that's what they are, and thankfully, they are a low salicylate food.

Black caraway: 2

Black caraway is categorized as high in salicylates, and we'll put it in a category below "very high." and give it a score of 2.

After some extensive digging we have been unable to find definitive information on the exact salicylate content, however we feel this spice should be limited or avoided altogether.

Blackberry: 1

Blackberries are rich in antioxidants, but they contain a very high amount of salicylates with over 1 mg per 100 g.

Blackcurrants: 1

Blackcurrants are usually cooked in savory or sweet dishes, and used to make syrup, preserves, or jam. Unfortunately they have a high level of salicylates, so mostly avoid or consume them minimally with caution, and be aware of their presence in other dishes.

Blue cheeses: 3

While most cheeses have negligible amounts of salicylates, blue cheese contains a moderate amount and should be limited in consumption despite containing more calcium than other types.

Blue fenugreek: 1

Blue fenugreek, widely used in Georgian cuisine, is very high in salicylates with at least 1 mg per 100 g.

Blueberries: 1

Blueberries are very high in salicylates, but they are also an extremely rich source of antioxidants which can lower the risk of serious health conditions like heart disease and cancer. Rather than avoid them altogether, consume on a limited basis.

Bok choi: 3

Also spelled as bok choy, our research has found that this leafy green vegetable has a moderate amount of salicylates, from .25 to .49 mg per 100 g.

A type of Chinese white cabbage in the cruciferous family, it's very high in vitamin C.

Borlotti beans: 1

See "Beans" for more information.

Bouillon: 1

It's difficult to rate store-bought bouillon and stocks as they typically contain a long list of ingredients that can vary greatly, but the most reliable lists rank them as high in salicylates.

Another negative, they contain flavor enhancers and other unhealthy ingredients like monosodium glutamate.

Boysenberry: 2

Boysenberries offer a slew of minerals like potassium, iron, calcium, and manganese, but they contain a very high level of salicylates, with at least 1 mg per 100 g.

Avoid or consume with caution in limited amounts.

Brandy: 2

Alcoholic beverages like beer, wine, and spirits such as rum and sherry tend to contain a high level of salicylates.

Champagne and sparkling wine are on the higher end, with Drambuie containing one of the highest levels for a liqueur. Dry, white wines have a lower amount while beer and ale can range anywhere from .32 to 1.26 per 100 g.

Of course, there are also the other negative health effects of alcohol to consider.

Brazil nuts: 3

Brazil nuts contain a moderate amount of salicylates, ranging from .25 to .49 mg per 100 g.

They are quite high in selenium which offers potent antioxidant properties to reduce inflammation and support heart health; however, it's important not to consume too many (which is difficult) as this quickly raises the salicylate content.

Bread: 3

Check ingredients individually. Here's why.

There are many different types of breads and when purchased at the supermarket, their ingredients can vary significantly which means you'll want to check each one in this guide.

The manufacturing process typically includes emulsifiers

and cutting oils along with other processing aids that can contain salicylates.

Many people with a salicylate sensitivity can tolerate most breads, but to be sure you might want to make your own using low-salicylate ingredients. Time-consuming, we know...

Broad beans: 1

Also known as Vicia Faba, see "Beans" for details.

Broccoli: 2

Broccoli offers a lot when it comes to nutrition, including more protein than most vegetables, along with fiber, vitamins C and K, but it contains reasonably high levels of salicylates depending on the source.

We've cautiously rated it as a "2" however you might find that you do okay with a small amount.

Brussels sprouts: 5

Brussels sprouts are low in salicylates and very rich in vitamin K as well as being an excellent source of vitamin C.

Buckwheat: 5

Buckwheat is a highly nutritious whole grain that's not only gluten-free, but very low in salicylates.

Butter: 5

All trustworthy lists consider butter to be very low in

salicylates; however, to avoid potential ill-effects that can come from hormones and additives, choose grass-fed, organic butter.

Cabbage: 5

Thankfully cabbage is low in salicylates as well as being versatile and cheap, even when purchasing organic. Plus, just a half-cup cooked provides about a third of your daily vitamin C requirements.

Cactus pear: 3

Also known as prickly pear and cactus fruit, cactus pears resemble pears in size and shape but it is not in the pear family.

There isn't a lot of information on them related to salicylates, a small clinical study published by medical analysis website eHealthMe found those who consumed it did not show an increase in salicylate levels in their bloodstream. Consume in limited amounts until you know how it will affect you.

Cactus pears have a high vitamin, mineral, and antioxidant content.

Cardamom: 2

Most spices are either high or very high in salicylates. Cardamom has been listed in both categories among reliable lists, making it best avoided or used in small amounts.

Carrot: 4

Fresh carrots contain a low to moderate amount of salicylates. Sources vary with some claiming there is under .25 mg per 100 g, But other sources categorize carrots as moderate in salicylates.

Cashew nuts: 4

Cashews have little to no salicylates and provide important nutrients, including plant protein and heart-healthy fats.

Cassava: 3

While there are some reliable lists that note cassava as a low salicylate food, others advise proceeding with caution as it is believed to be high in amygdalin which can cause a reaction in some who are salicylate sensitive.

Cassava is a root vegetable that is often used in flour form and that can make the salicylate content of store-bought treats high.

Cauliflower: 3

WebMD and a number of other reputable sites list cauliflower as having a high level of salicylates; however some rank it low or moderate.

The Cauliflower salicylate content has been shown in analysis to have approximately .25 mg per 100 g, but it does seem to vary.

This makes it difficult to score accurately, making it important to pay attention to how your body reacts to small amounts initially.

Celery: 5

Across the board, celery is listed as being a low salicylate food and it is filled with nutrients, including vitamins A, C, and K, calcium and potassium.

Cep mushrooms: 4

See "Mushrooms"

Chamomile and chamomile tea: 3

Herbal teas are often high in salicylates; however, chamomile has a moderately low amount according to several sites, with up to .25 mg per 100 g.

Due to inconsistencies we give this a moderate rating of 3.

Depending on your body chemistry you may be able to tolerate it when consumed in limited amounts.

Champagne: 1

Alcoholic beverages like beer, wine, and spirits such as rum and sherry tend to contain a high level of salicylates. And champagne and sparkling wine are considered to be on the higher end of the scale.

Unfortunately - high in salicylates,

Of course, there are also the other negative health effects of alcohol to consider.

Chard: 2

There isn't a lot of information about chard in relation to salicylates, but some sites do list it as having a high amount in addition to being very high in oxalates. It may be best to avoid, or at minimum proceed with caution.

Chard is also known by other names including Swiss chard, Roman kale, Sicilian beet, Chilean beet, silverbeet, leaf beat, spinach beet, and mangold.

Cheddar cheese: 5

See "Cheeses"

Cheese made from unpasteurized "raw" milk: 5

See "Cheeses"

Cheeses: 4

Other than blue cheeses, most cheeses are thought to be very low in salicylates. It contains high amounts of vitamins A and B-12 along with calcium, zinc, riboflavin, and phosphorus.

Choose cheeses made from 100 percent grass-fed animals for the highest level of nutrients and avoid processed types which may contain salicylates along with other potentially harmful ingredients.

Cherry: 2

Sour cherries have a moderate amount of salicylates, up to .49 mg per 100 g; however, fresh sweet cherries contain a high level, up to 1 mg per 100 g. Canned sweet cherries should be avoided as they are even higher in salicylates and often contain other unwanted ingredients.

Note that we have found some conflicting information, with some experts noting cherries in general (without indicating the type) as very high in salicylates. Based on this, you may want to avoid them altogether or choose only sour cherries, consumed in small amounts.

Chia, chia seeds: 1

While there is very little information on the amount of salicylates in chia seeds and they don't appear to have been tested in many studies, chia is a member of the mint family which contains a very high level of salicylates.

Those who are sensitive have reported adverse reactions to chia seeds, including ringing in the ears.

Chicken: 5

Chicken contains no or only trace amounts of salicylates, provided it is not processed, such as smoked and cured meats.

Choose fresh, organic options.

Chickpeas: 5

Chickpeas are not only low in salicylates, but these legumes are also an excellent source of fiber, iron, potassium, selenium, magnesium, and B vitamins to support heart health.

Chicory: 1

Avoid chicory as all our sources and lists rank it as very high in salicylates.

Chili pepper, red, fresh: 3

Hot chili peppers are very high in salicylates although the capsaicin they contain may reduce adverse effects.

Consume minimally until you know how your body will react.

Avoid sweet peppers which contain a high level of salicylates without the capsaicin.

Chives: 5

Chives are low in salicylates while being nutrient dense. They include the carotenoids lutein and zeaxanthin to support eye health and reduce the risk of macular degeneration.

Chocolate: 3

Chocolate has been reported by some with sensitivity to salicylates to have an adverse effect.

However, dark chocolate that is not made with raw sugar is considered to have a low amount by many reputable sites with reports that it is well-tolerated.

Cilantro: 2

Cilantro comes from the coriander plant. There is conflicting information as to how much salicylates it contains, although most reliable sources categorize it as "high" making it best to avoid or limit to very small amounts.

Cinnamon: 1

As with many spices, cinnamon is considered high in salicylates with at least 1 mg per 100 g.

Citrus fruits: 1

See the individual fruit as it varies as it varies depending on the type of citrus fruit. For example, lemons and limes are low or medium in salicylates; however, oranges are very high.

For this reason we've given citrus fruits a rating of 1 and encourage you to check each individual food.

Clover: 3

While there is not a lot of information on clover related to its salicylate content, some reliable sites list it as low in salicylates. This refers to clover in general, which can be red or white. The blossoms of red clover are known to contain salicylates but we have been unable to find analysis on the amount. That makes this wild veggie difficult to score, so once again, we ask you to proceed with caution.

Edible clover is a wild vegetable that's said to be highly nutritious though it's often referred to as a "weed."

As clover is a foraged food, if you choose to consume it, be sure that it is gathered from a pristine, clean source that has not been treated with chemicals.

Cloves: 1

Cloves are ranked anywhere from high to extremely high in salicylates.

Cocoa butter and cacao butter: 3

Chocolate, cocoa and cacao butters are thought to have low to moderate salicylates and are generally safe, including cocoa/cacao butter. The information is not definitive however and therefore we have given it a cautious 3 ranking.

Cocoa drinks, powder, etc: 1

See "Chocolate"

Coconut and coconut derivatives: 1

Fresh coconut, dried coconut (also referred to as desiccated), coconut milk and coconut water contain a moderate amount of salicylates, up to .49 mg per 100 g.

Coconut oil on the other hand thought to be very high in salicylates with over 1 mg per 100 g.

Coffee: 3

We know you want good information on coffee and

salicylates - the news though is mixed!

Decaf coffee contains negligible amounts of salicylates; however, regular coffee is considered to have a moderate level that ranges from .10 mg to .64 mg per 100 g depending on the brand.

If you must have a hot drink, coffee is better than most teas but to limit salicylates, go without the caffeine or mix half decaf and half regular.

Coriander: 2

See "Cilantro"

Corn salad, lamb's lettuce: 3

See "Lettuce"

Cornflakes: 4

Ready-to-eat cereals are generally low in salicylates, including cornflakes; however, they aren't the healthiest option, and other ingredients may well change the salicylate content.

Courgette: 1

There isn't a lot of information in relation to courgette and salicylates; however, some sources include it in the "high" or "very high" categories. Therefore we advise avoiding 'courgetti' and other courgette based dishes or consuming only in small amounts.

Crab: 5

Provided it's fresh and has not been preserved with sulfites, crab contains no or very little salicylates. It's packed with high levels of vitamin B12, selenium, and omega-3 fatty acids.

Cranberries and cranberry juice: 1

Cranberries, whether the fruit, juice, or canned in a sauce, are high in salicylates with at least 1 mg per 100g.

Crawfish: 5

Fish contains no to only trace amounts of salicylates according to most reliable sources.

Crayfish: 5

Fish contains no to only trace amounts of salicylates according to most reliable sources.

Cream cheeses: 5

See "Cheeses" or "Cream"

Cream: 5

Creams of all types are very low in salicylates, provided the ingredient list does not include additives.

It's high in calcium, but it's also high in fat which means it should be consumed in small amounts.

Generally, an organic grass-fed heavy cream is the better

choice as it is higher in nutrients like antioxidants and healthy fats.

Cress: 2

One of the oldest leafy greens known to humans, there is limited information available on the amount of salicylates in cress.

Watercress contains .49 to 1 mg, considered a "high" level, which is why we feel it's best to avoid or consume in small amounts until you know how it will affect you.

Cucumber: 2

Most reliable sources categorize cucumber as high in salicylates, with analysis sometimes showing it to have .78 mg per 100 g.

Cumin: 1

This is very much on our 'avoid list'.

Cumin seed contains a very high level of salicylates. According to NutritionFacts.org, eating a teaspoon of it is like taking a baby aspirin (one of the highest salicylate products you can consume)

Curry: 1

Curry is a popular Indian dish with a sauce seasoned with spices like turmeric, cumin, ginger, coriander, and chili pepper.

While ingredients may vary, as all recipes typically call for many spices that are very high in salicylates, it is best avoided.

Live Strong notes

Herbs and spices suspected to have high amounts of salicylates include curry, cumin powder, dill, oregano, hot paprika, rosemary, thyme, turmeric and vegemite.

Many of which are found in curries (but not vegemite!)

Dates: 1

Dates are high in natural sugars and said to contain a very high amount of salicylates. Avoid.

Note: Dried apricots and dates are often considered to be amongst the very highest salicylate foods.

Dextrose: 5

See "Sugar"

Dill: 1

An herb in the celery family, dill is extremely high in salicylates.

Dragon fruit: 1

Also referred to as white-fleshed pitahaya, dragon fruit is high in salicylates according to research published in the

International Archives of Allergy and Immunology.

Dried fruit: 1

Dried fruits such as apricots, raisins, and prunes contain high levels of salicylates.

Dried meat: 3

Dried meat that is unprocessed with no seasonings contains minimal or no salicylates; however, products like beef jerky typically contain additives and spices that make it high in salicylates.

This especially applies to store-bought products which are designed to have a longer shelf-life and therefore more potential salicylate-containing additives.

Dry-cured meats: 1

Curing is done using ingredients like sugar, salt, nitrate and/or nitrite for preservation, color, and flavor. We've found it hard to get specific, accurate information that we can reliably pass on about dry-cured meats, but given the ingredients and curing process varies, we believe that this alone makes it best treated with caution.

Duck: 5

See "Meat"

Eggs: 5

Both egg white and yolk are salicylate free; however,

according to research published in Food Additives & Contaminants:

Residues of salicylic acid in tissues and eggs may occur after drug administration or exposure of animals to feed material with high salicylate content.

The residue was found in very low concentrations with researchers noting that the eggs did not pose any risk to consumers sensitive to salicylates.

Still, we consider it important to buy organic, pasture-raised eggs which contain more nutrients, including omega-3 fatty acids, beta-carotene, and vitamins A, E, and D with less saturated fat and cholesterol.

Elderflower cordial: 1

Very high in salicylates, elderflower cordial is a soft drink that's made with the flowers of the European elder, typically combined with a solution of water and refined sugar.

Endive: 1

Our research shows that endive is very high in salicylates.

Espresso: 3

See "Coffee"

Fennel: 4

While the bulb of the fennel plant has a very low salicylate content, the leafy top is high in salicylates.

Stick to the bulb which has a fresh licorice flavor and crisp texture similar to celery, caramelising as it cooks for a sweeter taste.

Fenugreek: 1

Dried fenugreek contains a high level of salicylates with at least 1 mg per 100 g according to Molecular Nutrition & Food Research.

Feta cheese: 4

Most cheeses are thought to be very low in salicylates.

Choose cheeses made from 100 percent grass-fed animals for the highest level of nutrients and avoid processed types which may contain salicylates along with other potentially harmful ingredients.

Feta is also one of the lower-histamine cheeses so a good option for those with multiple intolerances.

Figs: 2

Fresh figs are low in salicylates with no more than .49 mg per 100 g; however, as with other dried fruits (see "Dried Fruits"), dried figs contain a high amount of salicylates.

While most people eat dried figs hence the 2 rating, however give the fresh version a go. It has a soft, jammy texture and is rich in vitamin A.

Fish: 5

Fish contains no to only trace amounts of salicylates according to most reliable sources.

Flaxseed (linseed): 2

We weren't able to find original research on salicylate levels in flaxseed that satisfied us to include in this dictionary.

Interestingly, some dermatologists treating patients with eczema have listed it as containing a moderate level and do not recommend it to those who are sensitive to salicylates. We have scored it accordingly.

Fructose: 1

Fructose is a fruit sugar that's often used in processed foods, we advise against consuming it.

Additionally, the peer-reviewed journal Alternative Medicine Review reports that it has caused chronic diarrhea and/or other bowel problems in some in addition to contributing to obesity and diabetes. We have struggled to source trustworthy information specifically available on fructose and salicylates, therefore we cannot provide a definitive rating above 1.

Game: 5

Fresh meat, including game, contains no salicylates. Avoid cured meats.

Garlic: 5

See "Broad-leaved garlic"

Ginger: 1

Ginger in any form, fresh, powder, or otherwise, contains a high level of salicylates with well over 1 mg per 100 g according to our best resources.

Goat's milk: 5

See "Milk"

Goji berry: 1

While there isn't any information available specifically related to the amount of salicylates in goji berries, berries in general contain a high content. This leads us to conclude that this superfood for some, is not a superfood for salicylate sufferers. So - it is best avoided or consumed in small amounts.

Goose (organic, pasture-raised): 5

See "Meat"

Gooseberry: 1

Gooseberries are thought to be high in salicylates.

Gouda cheese: 4

Most cheeses are thought to be very low in salicylates.

Choose cheeses made from 100 percent grass-fed animals for the highest level of nutrients and avoid processed types which may contain salicylates along with other potentially harmful ingredients.

Grapefruit: 2

Analysis from the Food Research Institute found no detectable salicylates in grapefruit; however, a number of reliable sources, including Millhouse Medical Centre and WebMD consider it to have a high amount. As a precautionary, we have scored it accordingly. Consume in moderation until you know how it will affect you.

Grapes: 2

Grapes vary in their salicylate content depending on the type which may be the reason for the conflicting information we've found among reliable sites.

Some of our favourite sources categorize grapes in general as "high" with numerous others rating red grapes in particular with a much higher content as compared to green, ranging between .49 mg and 1 mg per 100 g.

Our best advise based on available information is to choose green grapes and consume just a small amount until you know how they will affect you.

Green beans: 5

See "Beans"

Green peas: 4

Dried peas contain only trace amounts of salicylates while fresh green peas may have a low amount of up to .25 mg per 100 g.

Note that our score is based on dried peas or fresh green peas only as snow peas may contain a higher level.

As well as generally being thought to be low in salicylates, green peas are an excellent source of vitamin C as well as containing a good amount of protein, magnesium, iron, and fiber.

Green tea: 1

Most teas, including green tea according to WebMD, contain a very high level of salicylates.

Guava: 1

Whether fresh or canned, guava is very high in salicylates.

Ham (dried and cured): 1

While most meats do not contain salicylates, cured meats typically contain additives that make them best avoided. See "Dry-Cured Meats"

Hazelnuts: 3

According to multiple resources, hazelnuts have a low amount of salicylates,

Hazelnuts are an outstanding source of vitamin E and

magnesium, and they are high in calories. As we cannot be 100 percent sure based on available information as to the exact amount of salicylates in hazelnuts, consume in limited amounts or test carefully.

Hemp seeds (Cannabis sativa): 3

Most seeds contain a low to moderate amount of salicylates. We have scoured the Internet for information related to hemp seeds and were unable to find specific details.

Our research did yield some information on hemp seed oil which was shown to contain trace amounts of salicylates, reported in a lab analysis titled *The Composition of Hemp Seed Oil and Its Potential as an Important Source of Nutrition.*

Herbal tea: 1

Many if not most herbal teas are thought to contain a very high level of salicylates. See individual ingredients and teas for more details.

Honey: 1

High in salicylates with the exact level depending on the brand. Different honeys are thought to range between 2.5mg and over 10 mg of salicylates per 100 g, all considered high.

Horseradish: 4

Horseradish contains a low amount of salicylates, ranging from .15 to .25 mg per 100g.

Kale: 2

Kale is one of the reasons we wrote this book. Opinion differs significantly on kale and salicylates and that makes it a frustrating ingredient for sufferers of salicylate intolerance.

Guaranteeing the amount of salicylates in kale is impossible.

This popular superfood is ranked anywhere from low to high depending on which online source you consult, and for us, kale is always followed by a question mark.

As it is similar to chard, also known as Roman kale which is likely to contain a high level, we recommend avoiding or starting with a very limited amount until you know how your body will react.

Kefir: 5

Kefir is a fermented milk product.

As cow's milk, goat's milk, and other milk from animals are free of salicylates, provided it is made from one of these sources, we believe kefir should be as well. It's also loaded with probiotics that are good for your gut.

Kelp: 1

Kelp is a type of brown seaweed and as seaweed is high in salicylates, it should be avoided or consumed in very small amounts.

Kiwi: 2

Kiwi contains a moderate to high amount of salicylates depending on the analysis, making it best to err on the side of caution.

Kohlrabi: 4

A type of cultivar of wild cabbage in the same species as cabbage and Brussels sprouts, while there isn't a lot of information available on it in relation to salicylates, there are a few reliable sources ranking it low in salicylates.

Due to kohlrabi's relation to the other low salicylate vegetables, it is likely safe for sensitive individuals, however, consume in small amounts until you know how it will effect you.

Lamb: 5

See "Meat"

Lamb's lettuce/corn salad: 3

See "Lettuce"

Lard: 4

Lard is thought to be low in salicylates. It has about half as much saturated fat as butter, but double the amount found in olive oil. It is pork fat from the kidneys and back, and a good choice for cooking.

Leek: 5

Leeks are considered to be generally low in salicylates.

Lemon: 3

Most of our research has shown that lemons are low in salicylates, with up to .25 mg per 100 g. However, there are some sources that categorize this sour fruit as "moderate,".

Please note. There is anecdotal evidence from a number of sensitive individuals in the salicylate world reporting no negative effects from lemon or lemon juice. This conflicting information makes it difficult to accurate score lemons, hence the "3" rating.

Lentils: 5

Free or very low in salicylates, lentils are a reliable source of plant-based protein on a low-salicylate diet.

Lettuce: 4

The short answer is - it depends on the lettuce.

Iceberg is the most common type of lettuce and it is thought to contain only a negligible amount of salicylates.

Other lettuces can have higher levels of salicylates, such as lamb's lettuce and butterhead lettuce, which have a moderate level ranging from .25 to .49 mg per 100 g.

Lime: 5

Both limes and lime juice contain very low levels of salicylates according to multiple reliable sources.

Liquor: 2

Alcoholic beverages tend to contain a high level of salicylates.

Licorice: 1

Very high.

In a 1985 analysis of salicylates contents of foods by Swain et al, licorice was found to contain a very high level of salicylates, about 10 times higher than peppermints which are considered to be problematic for those who are sensitive.

Lobster: 5

Fish contains no to only trace amounts of salicylates according to most reliable sources.

Loganberry: 1

Like most berries, loganberries are thought to be high in salicylates.

Lychee: 3

Fresh lychee is moderately high in salicylates with up to .49 mg per 100 g. Consume in limited amounts, avoiding canned lychee which is often packed in heavy syrup.

Macadamia: 3

Macadamia nuts have a moderately high level of salicylates with just over .50 mg per 100 g. Some consumers have reported tolerating them in small amounts. They are calorie rich, high in healthy fats and nutrients.

Malt extract: 4

A rich source of soluble fiber, malt extract is also low in salicylates.

Malt: 4

The germinated cereal grain dried in a process called "malting" is low in salicylates, but if you're on a gluten-free diet you'll want to avoid it.

Maltodextrin: 3

Not the best choice for those following a more natural, whole food diet as it's often derived from GMO corn, though it is typically low in salicylates.

See "Sweeteners"

Mandarin orange: 2

Fresh mandarin is moderately high in salicylates with potentially over .5 mg per As with everything on a low-salicylate diet, proceed with caution if you are going to consume mandarin orange and test carefully first.

Mango: 3

Opinion varies between the major sites. Proceed with caution if you are highly sensitive. While high in vitamins A and C, it also contains a high level of natural fruit sugars.

Maple syrup: 4

Maple syrup is thought to be low in salicylates (but high in sugar).

Margarine: 1

Margarine and salicylates is a complicated relationship.

As with other intolerances such as histamine intolerance, some foods contain salicylate and some foods cause a salicylate reaction. Margarine falls in that category. We can't vouch for the exact levels of salicylates in an individual margarine, however margarine in general is thought to contain preservatives that can mimic salicylates or cause salicylate flare-ups.

This is in addition to trans fats which are associated with an increased risk of heart disease and other, sometimes numerous, ingredients.

Marrow: 3

Marrow ranges from low to moderate depending on the source, containing over .15 mg per 100g. As it is categorized as moderate by some reliable sources, it's best to proceed with caution.

Mascarpone cheese: 4

Most cheeses are thought to be very low in salicylates.

Choose mascarpone made from 100 percent grass-fed animals for the highest level of nutrients and avoid processed types which may contain salicylates along with other potentially harmful ingredients.

Mate tea: 1

Mate, like most teas, is high in salicylates.

Meat: 4

Meat is generally salicylate free but avoid liver and all processed meats. To support general health, look for organic, grass-fed meats to avoid unwanted hormones and chemicals.

Melon: 2

It all depends on what type of melon. The amount of salicylates in this fruit depends on the type of melon, with most containing a moderate to high amount.

Watermelon was analyzed to contain moderate amounts of salicylates while other melons such as cantaloupe (also known as rock-melon) were shown to have a much higher level.

Milk: 5

Most dairy products typically have little or no salicylates, including animal milks of all types like goat's and cow's milk.

Important note: Be aware that non-animal milks often used in trendy coffee shops like almond and coconut milk have a high level of salicylates.

Millet: 5

Millet contains negligible amounts of salicylates.

Mincemeat: 1

Mincemeat may contain some beef which is typically salicylate free, but it's generally a mixture of ingredients that are high in salicylates such as spices, dried fruit, and distilled spirits.

Mint: 1

Mint, whether the herb, peppermint candy or in chewing gum, is high in salicylates.

Morel: 3

There is no information on the content of salicylates in morel or truffles available that we were able to find, making it impossible to accurately categorize it.

Fresh mushrooms do have a low level at about .24 mg per 100 g which may be an indication but proceed with caution if you're sensitive.

Morello cherries: 4

Sour canned morello cherries have a low amount of

salicylates at less than .25 mg per 100 mg.

Mozzarella cheese: 4

"Most cheeses are thought to be very low in salicylates.

Choose cheeses made from 100 percent grass-fed animals for the highest level of nutrients and avoid processed types which may contain salicylates along with other potentially harmful ingredients."

Mulberry: 1

As a berry, mulberries have a high level of salicylates with .76 mg per 100 g.

Mungbeans (germinated, sprouting): 5

Mungbeans are free of salicylates.

Mushrooms: 4

Mushrooms of all types have a low amount of salicylates, with analysis showing a range of up to but not over .25 g per 100 g.

Mustard and mustard seeds: 1

Mustard and mustard seeds are very high in salicylates.

Napa cabbage: 5

Thankfully cabbage is thought to be low in salicylates as well as being versatile and cheap, even when purchasing organic. Plus, just a half-cup cooked provides about a third of your daily vitamin C requirements.

Nectarine: 2

Nectarine is another fruit that tends to be quite high in salicylates. Not all sources agree on the exact levels, but they do tend to agree that this is a fruit to approach with caution.

Nettle tea: 3

There have not been many studies looking at the amount of salicylates in nettle leaves, although some reports do indicate that it is very low.

Frustratingly, as we cannot be sure, we've ranked it in the middle, meaning consume a small amount until you know how it will affect you. This is one of the foods and ingredients we are hoping to update on this list as more research becomes available.

Nori seaweed: 1

Seaweed, including Nori seaweed, is very high in salicylates.

Nutmeg: 1

Very high in salicylates as with most spices, nutmeg has been analyzed to contain 2.4 mg per 100 g.

That said, as with most spices, you may not be consuming many grams of nutmeg, but proceed with caution.

Nuts: 1

See the individual nut for details.

We've ranked nuts in general as a "1" as they can be very low or high depending on the particular type.

Oats: 5

Oats contain negligible amounts of salicylates, if any.

Olive oil: 2

Olive oil is made from olives which can be high in salicylates depending on the type. Olive oil is similarly thought to be on the highish range of salicylate content.

Olives: 2

While some reliable sources list olives in general as potentially being high in salicylates, black olives are a bit lower, coming in at .34 mg per 100 g.

Green olives tend to test much higher at over 1 mg per 100 g.

Onion: 3

There is plenty of debate about onions and salicylates. Most sources seem to agree that the levels of salicylates are not extremely high, but they still need to be approached with caution.

Fresh onions according to multiple trustworthy analyses, including a study published in the *Journal of the American Dietetic Association* Vol. 85:8 1985, have been found to contain .16 mg to .18 mg of salicylates per 100 g, placing them in the "low level" category.

However, other food lists and studies believe salicylate levels in onions are higher.

Onions are rich in powerful antioxidants and other compounds known to fight inflammation, reduce triglycerides and cholesterol levels which can lower heart disease risk, so they are something that you may want to try and retain on your low salicylate diet.

Orange: 1

Oranges are thought to contain a high level of salicylates

Oregano: 1

Spices in general tend to be high in salicylates. Oregano is another spice that is high in salicylates.

Ostrich: 5

Despite coming from a bird, ostrich tastes more like premium beef and is rich in iron while lower in fat and cholesterol as well as being free from salicylates.

For more information, see "Meat"

Oysters: 5

See "Bivalves"

Papaya: 5

Papaya is one of the lowest salicylate fruits. We even considered putting a papaya on the cover of this food dictionary.

It is low in salicylates but loaded with nutrients. It's particularly rich in vitamin A, C, and antioxidants to help reduce the risk of cancer.

Parsley: 2

This is one where emerging research is changing the way we think about an ingredient.

Parsley was initially believed to be low in salicylates but reliable sources have noted recent research revealing the opposite to be true.

This has led to a lot of conflicting information, with it ranked as low, moderate, or high. Frustrating, we know, but that's why this food dictionary is important, as if you relied on one list you wouldn't know this.

Consider this when making your decision whether or not to include it in your diet, consuming small amounts before you know how your body will react.

Parsnip: 3

Parsnip contains a moderate amount of salicylates.

Passion fruit: 2

While passion fruit is often rated as high in salicylates, some food lists demur and say it is lower. Most fruits do contain a high amount, so we've decided to err on the side of caution and give it a cautious '2' rating.

Peach: 2

Both fresh and canned peaches contain a moderately high amount of salicylates.

Peanuts: 1

Peanuts are thought to be very high in salicylates. One to avoid on a low salicylate diet.

Web MD notes; Cereals that contain almonds or peanuts are high in salicylates and should be avoided.

The website drugs.com also notes peanuts are high in salicylates.

Naturally Savvy notes the following food products may also contain salicylates;

Nuts such as pine nuts, peanuts, pistachios, and almonds

Pear: 4

Pears are another fruit we considered putting on the front cover of this food dictionary. They can be very low in salicylates but only under certain conditions.

Peeling your pear is key.

If you peel a pear before eating it, it will have no salicylates or only a trace amount; however, unpeeled pears may be quite high in salicylates.

Peas (green): 4

See "Green peas"

Pea shoots/pea sprouts: 1

The latest food chemical chart from Royal Prince Alfred Hospital's Allergy Unit (RPAH), the world's leading allergy unit in terms of food chemicals like salicylates, notes that they contain a high amount.

This is a shame because they can be very healthy in other aspects and even histamine-lowering too, but as such proceed with great caution.

There isn't, however, a lot of information on pea shoots, also called pea sprouts, in relation to salicylates, so we await further research.

Peppermint tea: 1

As an herbal tea, peppermint also contains a high level of salicylates.

Pickled foods: 1

Royal Prince Alfred Hospital's Allergy Unit (RPAH), the world's leading allergy unit in terms of food chemicals like salicylates, (mentioned above) lists all pickled foods, including pickles, pickled cucumber, pickled olives, and pickled onions as very high in salicylates.

Pineapple: 1

Very high in salicylates.

Pistachio: 2

Pistachio nuts are thought to contain quite a high amount of salicylates - often over .5 mg per 100 g.

As per *Healthline*, they are rich in healthy fats, antioxidants, protein, and various nutrients like vitamin B6.

Unless you're very sensitive you may be able to consume a very limited amount (one to three pistachios) without negative effects. But one to three pistachios doesn't sound much fun - sorry!

Plum: 2

Plums are difficult to score. We advise avoiding canned plums and if you decide to eat fresh plums, start with a small amount until you know how your body will react.

Fresh plums are thought to be lower in salicylates than canned plums, but the salicylate community is divided on whether plums in general are low or high in salicylates.

Pomegranate: 2

Unfortunately, after extensive research we found most trustworthy sites categorize pomegranates as high in salicylates.

It is though, another difficult fruit to score, as analysis by the ADA finding pomegranates to be very low in salicylates.

Who's right then? Unfortunately, as always this is an area

where you will have to work out your own tolerance level to pomegranate.

Poppy seeds: 5

Negligible amount of salicylates.

Pork: 5

See "Meat"

Potato: 3

The next time you make mashed potatoes, use your peeler to avoid salicylates. Peeled white potatoes are thought to be free of salicylates while unpeeled white potatoes contain a low amount, up to .25 mg per 100g.

So potatoes are a bit like pears. Potato and pear salad anyone? Ignore us, let's continue.

Be aware that not all potatoes are created equal.

Red potatoes and yellow sweet potatoes have a moderate amount of salicylates, and sweet potatoes are thought to be high in salicylates as well as oxalates.

In summary, if you're not ultra-sensitive to salicylates but want to maximize nutrition choose unpeeled white potatoes. Te skin offers a good amount of fiber, B vitamins, vitamin C, and other beneficial nutrients. If you are ultra-sensitive - peel 'em.

Poultry: 1

See "Meat"

Prawn: 1

See "Fish" while keeping in mind that fried versions may contain salicylates and other ingredients that do not support optimal health. Prawns are the one fish noted by the *Food Can Make You Ill* website to avoid.

Processed cheese: 4

Most cheeses are thought to be very low in salicylates.

But keep in mind that processed cheese is high in sodium and saturated fat along with unhealthy additives. Regular consumption can lead to obesity and hypertension, the reason for our ranking.

Prune: 1

Thought to be extremely high in salicylates. Indeed, there are possibly more salicylates in prunes than any other fruit.

The website Allergenics notes;

Dried fruits such as apricots, raisins, dates and prunes have extremely high levels.

Pulses: 1-5

Pulses include common beans, peas, chickpeas, fava beans, and lentils, all of which vary in salicylates, from a low amount in chickpeas to a high level in fava beans.

Check the individual pulse for details.

Pumpkin seed oil:

See "Pumpkin seeds"

Pumpkin seeds: 3

Pumpkin seeds are thought to contain a moderate amount of salicylates.

Pumpkin: 4

Most reliable sources consider fresh and canned pumpkin to be low in salicylates, with analysis revealing .12 mg per 100 mg. However, some list pumpkin as containing a moderate level of salicylates.

If you tolerate pumpkin well, you'll benefit from many nutrients like vitamins A, C, manganese, folate, potassium, calcium, and some of the B vitamins.

Quinoa: 5

Quinoa is not only a whole protein, it's versatile gluten-free and salicylate-free seed that can be ground into a flour, used whole in stews, or even as a breakfast cereal.

Rabbit: 5

See "Meats"

Raclette cheese: 5

Most cheeses are thought to be very low in salicylates.

Choose cheeses made from 100 percent grass-fed animals for the highest level of nutrients and avoid processed types which may contain salicylates along with other potentially harmful ingredients.

Radish: 1

High in salicylates.

Raisins: 1

Raisins are very high in salicylates, with some of the highest levels of any fruit analyzed by the American Dietetic Association.

Rapeseed/canola oil: 4

Unlike peanut oil and olive oil, canola oil contains only a negligible amount of salicylates.

Known as canola oil in the U.S. and rapeseed oil in many other countries.

However, while some can tolerate canola oil well, it can lead to inflammation in others. A number of animal studies have linked it to oxidative stress and increased inflammation. An Australian study published in *Lipids in Health and Disease* found that rats fed a diet that included 10 percent canola oil experienced increases in LDL ("bad") cholesterol and decreases in multiple antioxidants.

The website *Food Can Make You Ill* provides a comprehensive breakdown of an Australian study (Anne R Swain et al.

Salicylates in Food. Journal of the American Dietetic Association Vol. 85:8 1985). It notes;

Margarine and processed rapeseed (canola), safflower, soya bean, sunflower oils although low in salicylate are likely to contain preservatives that may mimic salicylate reactions and are best avoided.

Raspberry: 1

Raspberries are a significant source of salicylates.

The website Allergy Link puts raspberries on its list of Salicylate containing foods and they should be treated with caution.

Raw milk: 5

Most dairy products typically have little or no salicylates, including animal milks of all types like goat's and cow's milk.

Important note: Be aware that non-animal milks often used in trendy coffee shops like almond and coconut milk have a high level of salicylates.

Raw milk has been shown to provide greater bioavailable nutrients than pasteurized versions along with a wide range of beneficial probiotics and enzymes.

Red cabbage: 5

Thankfully cabbage is thought to be low in salicylates as well as being versatile and cheap, even when purchasing organic. Plus, just a half-cup cooked provides about a third of your daily vitamin C requirements.

Red wine vinegar: 1

High in salicylates with up to 1 mg per 100 mg.

Redcurrants: 1

Very high in salicylates. Currants are among the highest salicylate foods.

Rhubarb: 4

Fresh rhubarb is thought to be low in salicylates.

The website *Food Can Make You Ill* provides a comprehensive breakdown of an Australian study (Anne R Swain et al. Salicylates in Food. Journal of the American Dietetic Association Vol. 85:8 1985). It includes rhubarb in its 'low' list.

Rice: 5

Rice of all types is thought to contain trace amounts of salicylates.

Rice cakes: 3

While rice contains very little or no salicylates, rice cakes typically contain other ingredients that are not or that may have a negative impact on health like sugars and artificial colorings.

Look for non-GMO, organic options and check individual ingredients.

Rice milk: 4

Generally rice milk is low in salicylates; however, you'll need to check the individual ingredients with the fewer the better. For example, some include canola, safflower or sunflower oils, flavorings, and other additives.

Important note: Be aware that non-animal milks often used in coffee shops like almond and coconut milk have a high level of salicylates. Rice milk we hope will work better for you, but can be higher in sugar.

Rice noodles: 4

Typically low in salicylates, but again, it's important to check individual ingredients.

Ricotta cheese: 5

Most cheeses are thought to be very low in salicylates.

Choose ricotta cheese made from 100 percent grass-fed animals for the highest level of nutrients and avoid processed types which may contain salicylates along with other potentially harmful ingredients.

Rooibos tea:1

Very high in salicylates.

Roquefort cheese: 5

Most cheeses are thought to be very low in salicylates.

Choose roquefort made from 100 percent grass-fed animals for the highest level of nutrients and avoid processed types which may contain salicylates along with other potentially harmful ingredients.

Rosemary: 1

Very high in salicylates.

Rum: 2

Alcoholic beverages like beer, wine, and spirits such as rum and sherry tend to contain a high level of salicylates.

Rye: 5

Rye contains little if any salicylates; however, if you are gluten intolerant, be aware that it is not gluten-free.

Sage: 1

High in salicylates.

Salami: 1

See "Dry-cured meats"

Salmon: 5

Fish contains no to only trace amounts of salicylates according to most reliable sources.

Sauerkraut: 1

Very high in salicylates. Also very high in histamine - those with multiple food sensitivities should avoid.

Sausage (all types): 1

While most meats are free of salicylates, sausage contains spices and other flavorings that make it best to avoid for those who are sensitive.

Savoy cabbage: 5

Thankfully cabbage is thought to be low in salicylates as well as being versatile and cheap, even when purchasing organic. Plus, just a half-cup cooked provides about a third of your daily vitamin C requirements. As always test carefully, but cabbage is one of our low-salicylate staples.

Schnapps: 2

Alcoholic beverages tend to contain a high level of salicylates. See "alcohol" for more details.

Seafood: 5

Fish contains no to only trace amounts of salicylates according to most reliable sources.

Seaweed: 1

Very high in salicylates.

Sesame: 3

There is a distinction here between sesame seeds and sesame oil.

Sesame seeds are thought to be lowish in salicylates. However, sesame oil contains a higher amount and should be limited or avoided.

Sheep's milk: 5

See "Milk" - generally a good option.

Shellfish: 5

Fish is normally fine. See "Fish" and "Bivalves" and the note below under "Shrimp"

Shrimp: 5

Be aware that canned shrimp and/or shrimp sprayed with sulfites will contain a moderate to high amount of salicylates. Avoid fried shrimp which typically contain a high level. See "Prawns" for another important note.

Smoked meat: 1

While meats in general are free of salicylates, smoked meats typically contain a higher amount.

Snow peas: 3

See "Green peas"

Soft cheese: 5

Most cheeses are thought to be very low in salicylates.

Choose cheeses made from 100 percent grass-fed animals for the highest level of nutrients and avoid processed types which may contain salicylates along with other potentially harmful ingredients.

Sour Cream: 4

Sour cream is low in salicylates; however, it's important to check for any added ingredients that may contain a higher level.

Soy (including soy beans and soy flour): 1

An excellent source of protein that makes it especially ideal for anyone on a plant-based diet, soy contains a negligible amount of salicylates.

Soy sauce: 4

Provided it is free of spices and other additives, soy sauce is low in salicylates.

Sparkling wine: 1

Alcoholic beverages tend to contain a high level of salicylates. See "alcohol" for more details. Sparkling wine is thought by some to be particularly high hence the "1" rating.

Spelt: 5

Spelt is low in salicylates and while it's technically a type of wheat, this is an ancient form that many people on gluten-free diets can tolerate.

Spinach: 3

Fresh spinach contains a moderately high level of salicylates. However, there is a hack that some people swear by.

If you like spinach and want to enjoy its many beneficial nutrients with high amounts of carotenoids and a rich amount of vitamins A, C, K, iron, and potassium, try it frozen.

Frozen spinach is thought to possibly be better tolerated on a low-salicylate diet, but must be tested carefully.

Spirits: 2

Alcoholic beverages tend to contain a high level of salicylates. See "alcohol" for more details."

Stevia: 3

A processed sugar substitute, Stevia is made from the leaf of a plant and is in the Asteraceae family. It does not appear to have been tested; however, most salicylate sensitive people can tolerate it. Be cautious until you know how your body will react. If you have an allergy to ragweed, it may not be the best choice.

Stinging nettle: 1

There is very little information on the amount of salicylates in stinging nettle.

Some anecdotally report that it is likely to contain at least some salicylates while others note that it is free of the compound, making it impossible to score accurately.

Strawberry: 1

Very high in salicylates.

Sugar: 5

Standard white sugar is free of salicylates; however it's believed to be a big contributor to the obesity epidemic and can increase the risk of developing many other health conditions. Lecture over.

Sunflower oil: 1

Negligible amount of salicylates. There's a big *but* coming though.

The website *Food Can Make You Ill* notes;

Margarine and processed rapeseed (canola), safflower, soya bean, sunflower oils although low in salicylate are likely to contain preservatives that may mimic salicylate reactions and are best avoided.

Sunflower seeds: 4

Very low amount of salicylates.

Sweet corn: 3

Fresh sweet corn is low in salicylates; however, canned sweet corn may contain a moderate amount, hence the "3" rating.

Sweet potato: 2

Yellow sweet potatoes have a moderate amount of salicylates, and sweet potatoes are thought to be high in salicylates as well as oxalates. Those with multiple food sensitivities should avoid.

Tea, black: 1

Very high in salicylates.

Thyme: 1

Very high in salicylates.

Tomato: 2

Fresh tomato seems to be lower than canned tomatoes, tomato paste, and tomato sauce in terms of salicylates. And then there's a distinction between raw tomato and cooked tomato.

The website Allergenics notes;

Salicylates are found in plants, and in higher concentrations in plants that are concentrated by drying or juicing or making into sauces pastes or jams. So while tomatoes may be high in salicylates, tomato paste will be higher. Raw tomatoes will have higher levels than cooked tomatoes though- it's tricky!

Trout: 5

Fish contains no to only trace amounts of salicylates according to most reliable sources.

Tuna: 5

Fish contains no to only trace amounts of salicylates according to most reliable sources. Canned tuna often contains high mercury levels.

Turkey: 5

See "Meat"

Turmeric:

Thought to be very high in salicylates.

Turnip: 4

Some conflicting information, categorized as low to moderate in salicylates depending on the source.

Venison: 5

See "Meat"

Vinegar, balsamic: 1

We believe to be moderate to high in salicylates.

However Live Strong notes;

Fennel, vinegar and soy sauce contain moderate amounts

Vinegar, distilled white: 1

High in salicylates.

The website Allergenics notes;

Sauces and Condiments: most commercial or store-bought gravies, sauces and pastes (eg. tomato paste, worcester sauce, gravy mix), jams, marmalades, fruit/mint/honey flavouring, chewing gum, white and cider vinegars

However Live Strong notes;

Fennel, vinegar and soy sauce contain moderate amounts

Walnut: 3

There is a bit of a debate as to the amount of salicylates in walnuts, with some analysis showing high levels of salicylates, and other reliable sources listing them as "moderate" in salicylates.

Whether high or moderate, it seems walnut does contain levels of salicylates that require a cautious approach. They are also very high in histamine - those with multiple food sensitivities should avoid.

Watercress: 2

Watercress has a fairly high amount of salicylates.

Watermelon: 3

Watermelon was analyzed to contain moderate amounts of salicylates while other melons such as cantaloupe (also known as rock-melon) were shown to have a much higher level.

There is some debate over watermelon so approach cautiously. As it is such a close call, there is inconsistency in site ratings, listed as either moderate or high depending on the source.

Wheat: 4

The grain wheat itself is free of salicylates; however, as it's not eaten on its own when made into a bread you'll need to consider the other ingredients. Additionally, many find eliminating gluten from their diet can improve their overall well-being.

Wheat germ: 5

Part of a wheat kernel that helps the plant reproduce, wheat germ is free of salicylate. Refer to "Wheat" for more details.

White button mushroom: 4

See "Mushrooms"

Wild rice: 5

Generally fine. See "Rice:

Wine: 2

Alcoholic beverages tend to contain a high level of salicylates. See "alcohol" for more details.

Yam: 3

See "Potatoes" (yam is of the potato family)

Yogurt/Yoghurt: 5

Yogurt is a calcium-rich food that is free of salicylates.

However, for optimal health avoid versions with sugars and additives, ideally choosing plain yogurt mixed with a low-salicylate fruit or nuts for added flavor and crunch.

Zucchini: 1

High in salicylates. Also known as courgettes. Often makes lists of the highest salicylate content in vegetables alongside chicory, endive, and peppers.

HOUSEHOLD CLEANING PRODUCTS, CHEMICALS, PERSONAL CARE ITEMS AND MEDICINES

Salicylates are, frustratingly, everywhere. They are not only found in food and drink items, but in household cleaning products, chemicals, personal care items such as shampoos, in perfumes, and in some medicines, particularly aspirin.

If you're taking prescription medications, your healthcare provider can advise you on any salicylates in them.

The excellent website *Allergy Link* provides a list of what to watch out:

- fragrances
- perfumes
- shampoos
- conditioners
- herbal remedies
- lipsticks

- lotions
- skin cleansers
- mouthwash
- toothpaste (mint)
- shaving cream
- sunscreens
- tanning lotions
- muscle pain ointments

We've found that the lists of individual ingredients that may cause sensitivities are fairly long and involved, and unfortunately you may have carry out your own individual research on each product. As a rule we have found that natural products with less ingredients are normally a better option.

Additionally, as we've mentioned, many processed foods have chemical additives that can contain salicylates so it's best to look out for those, and track your own progress with foods, personal care products, cleaning products and so on.